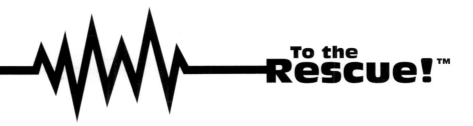

Ambulances

Joanne Randolph

PowerKiDS
press.
New York

For Riley, Deming, and Hannah

Published in 2008 by The Rosen Publishing Group, Inc.
29 East 21st Street, New York, NY 10010

First Edition

Book Design: Greg Tucker
Photo Researcher: Nicole Pristash

Photo Credits: Cover, pp. 7, 11, 13, 15, 19, 21, 24 (top left), 24 (bottom left), 24 (bottom right) Shutterstock.com; p. 5 © www.iStockphoto.com/Hazlan Abdul Hakim; p. 9 © www.iStockphoto.com/Nancy Louie; p. 17, 24 (top right) © www.iStockphoto.com/David Dea; p. 23 © www.iStockphoto.com/Tana Minnick.

Library of Congress Cataloging-in-Publication Data

Randolph, Joanne.
  Ambulances / Joanne Randolph. — 1st ed.
      p. cm. — (To the rescue!)
  Includes index.
  ISBN 978-1-4042-4150-3 (library binding)
  1. Ambulances—Juvenile literature. 2. Emergency medicine—Juvenile literature. I. Title.
  TL235.8.R36 2008
  362.18'8—dc22

                                    2007021210

Manufactured in the United States of America

Contents

Ambulances save people's lives every day.

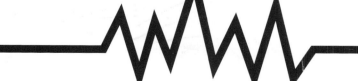

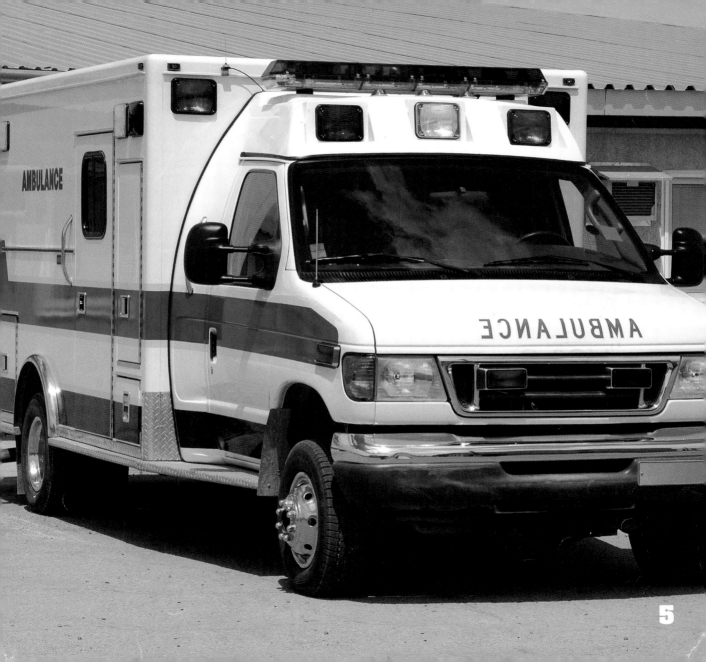

The people who drive
ambulances are called EMTs
or **paramedics**.

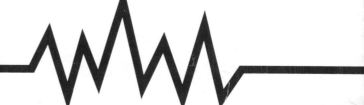

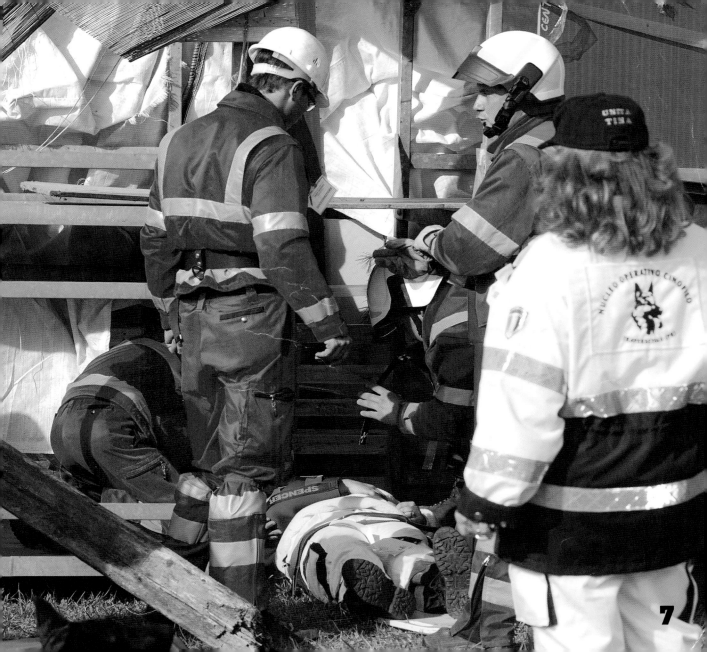

EMTs and paramedics help people who are sick or hurt.

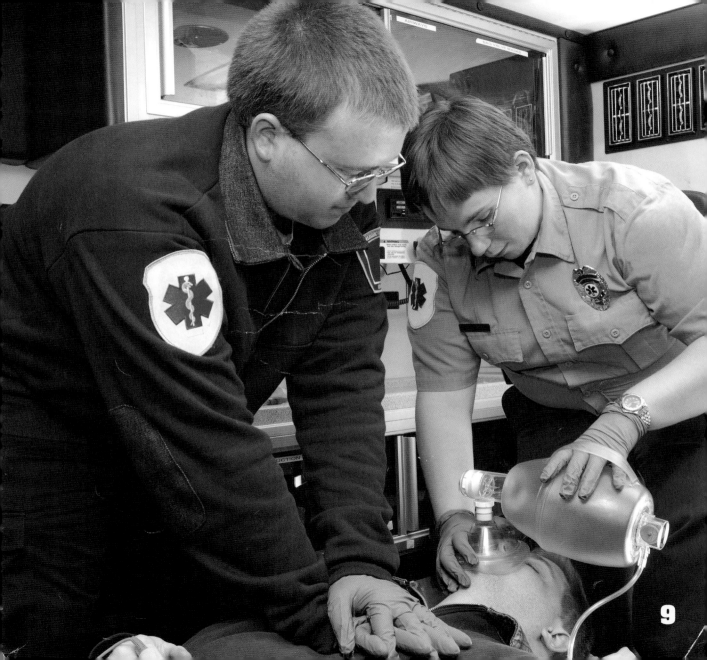

Ambulances have lights on top. The lights are turned on when an ambulance is on its way to help someone.

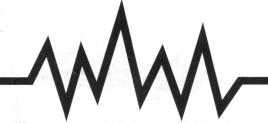

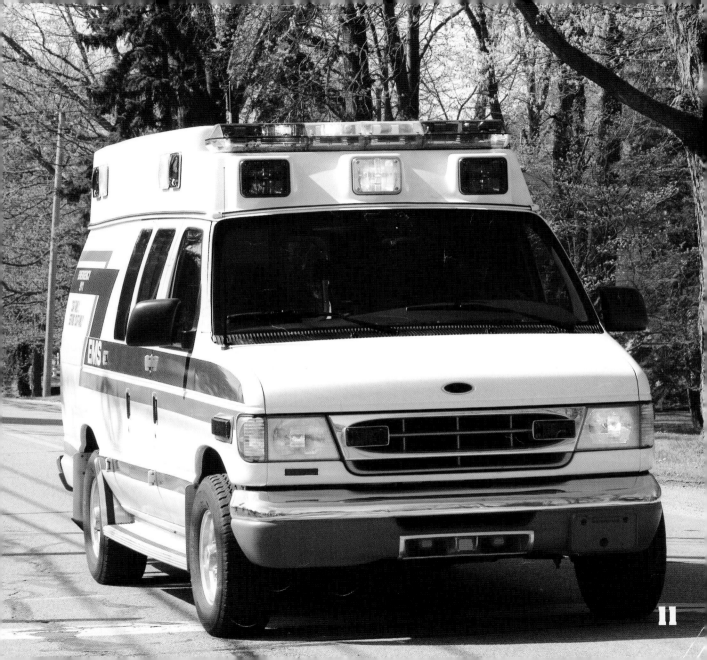

Sick people are put on a **stretcher** to ride in the back of the ambulance.

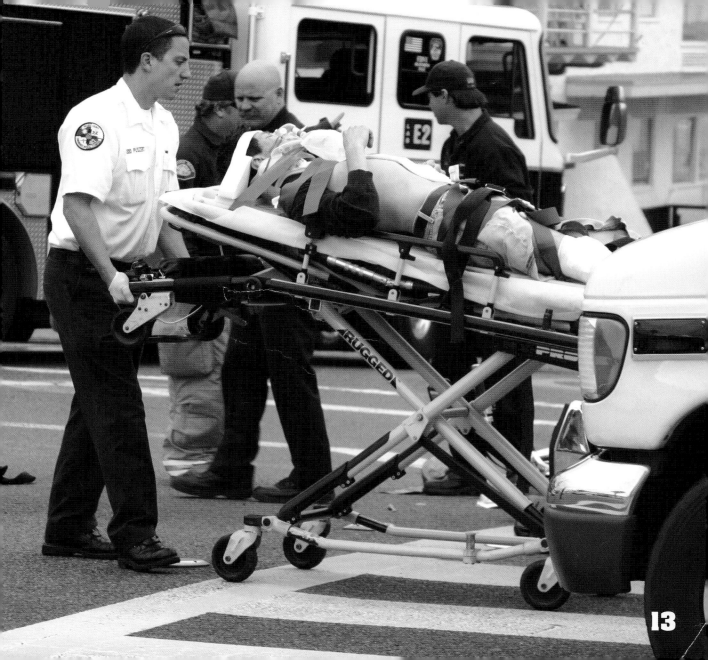

This is the inside of an ambulance. It has everything EMTs and paramedics need to do their job.

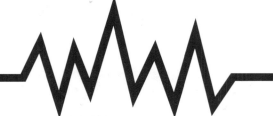

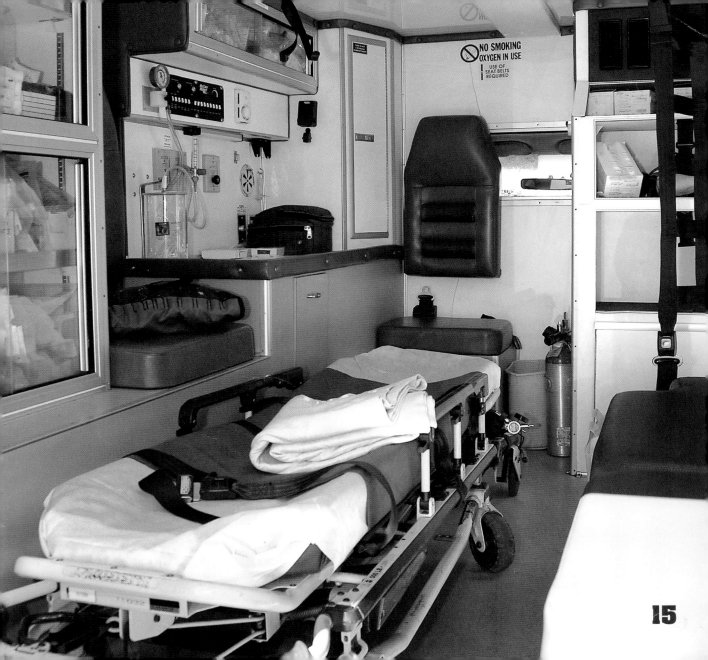

NO SMOKING
OXYGEN IN USE

USE OF
SEAT BELTS
REQUIRED

15

Ambulances bring people to the **hospital**.

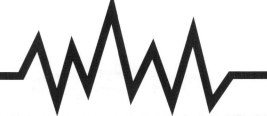

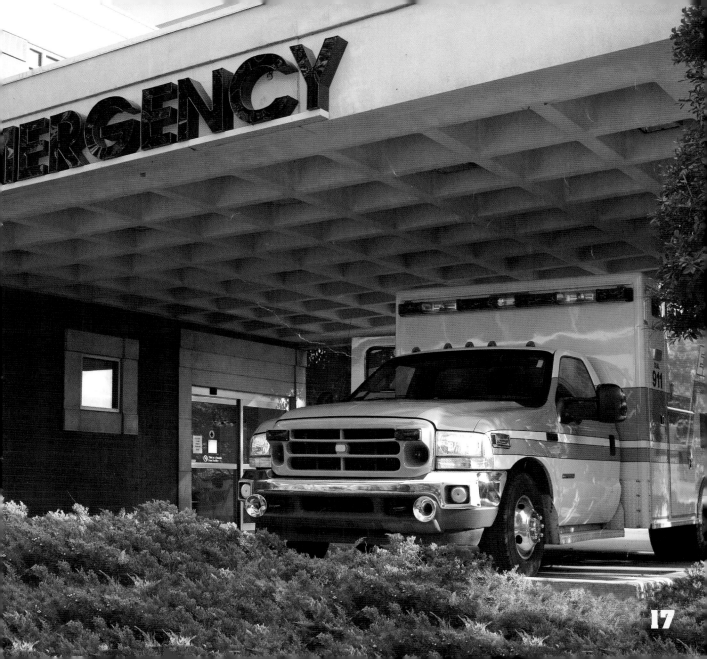

Ambulances are called to help out after a **car crash**.

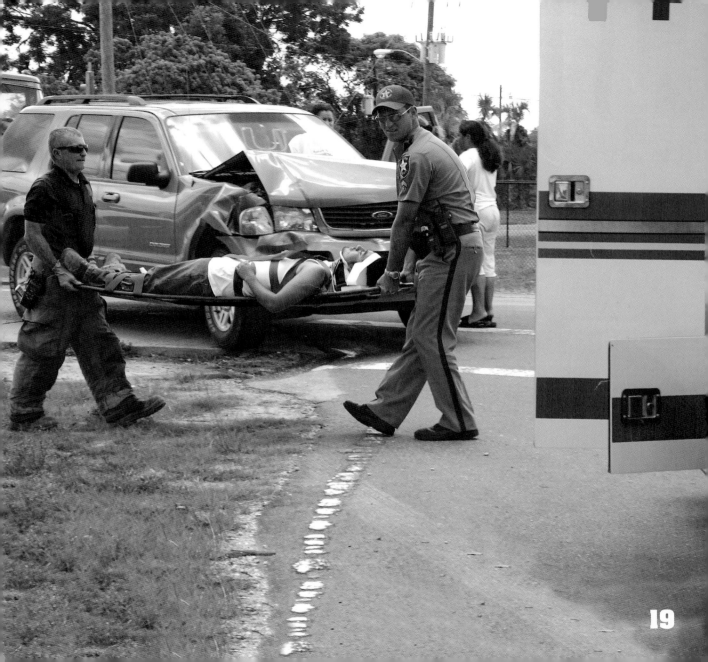

Ambulances help out anywhere someone could be hurt or sick.

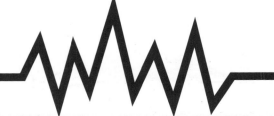

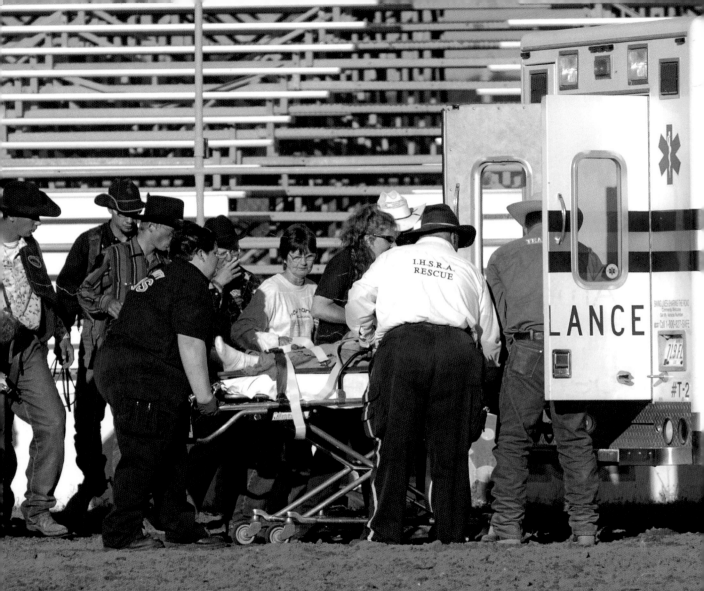

Thank goodness there are ambulances ready to help people in need!

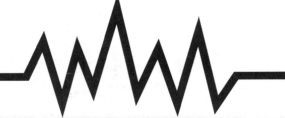

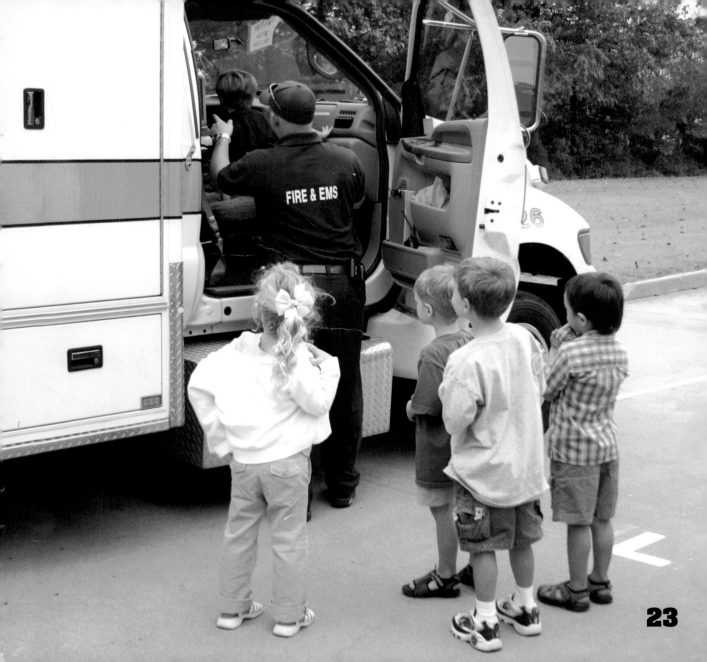

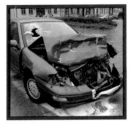

car crash

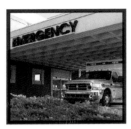

hospital

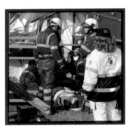

paramedics

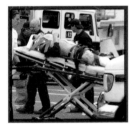

stretcher

Index

Web Sites

Due to the changing nature of Internet links, PowerKids Press has developed an online list of Web sites related to the subject of this book. This site is updated regularly. Please use this link to access the list:
www.powerkidslinks.com/ttr/ambul/